Dr Dawn's Guide to Y

ch of the

wn Harper is a GP based in Gloucestershire, working date s surgery in Stroud. She has been working as a media doctor for nearly ten years. Dawn is best known as one of the presenters on Channel 4's award-winning programme *Embarrassing Bodies*, which has run for seven series and two years ago celebrated its hundredth episode. Spin-offs have included *Embarrassing Fat Bodies*, *Embarrassing Teen Bodies* and *Embarrassing Bodies: Live from the clinic*.

Dawn is the presenter of Channel 4's series *Born Naughty?*, one of the doctors on ITV1's *This Morning* and the resident GP on the health hour on LBC radio. She writes for a variety of publications, including *Healthspan*, *Healthy Food Guide* and *NetDoctor*. Her first book, *Dr Dawn's Health Check*, was published by Mitchell Beazley. *Dr Dawn's Guide to Your Baby's First Year* is one of ten Dr Dawn Guides published by Sheldon Press in 2015 and 2016. Dawn qualified at London University in 1987. When not working, she is a keen cyclist and an enthusiastic supporter of children's charities. She is also a mother of three. Her website is at <www.drdawn.com>. Follow her on Twitter @drdawnharper.

Overcoming Common Problems Series

Selected titles

A full list of titles is available from Sheldon Press,
36 Causton Street, London SW1P 4ST and on our website at
www.sheldonpress.co.uk

Beating Insomnia: Without really trying
Dr Tim Cantopher

Birth Over 35
Sheila Kitzinger

Breast Cancer: Your treatment choices
Dr Terry Priestman

The Chronic Fatigue Healing Diet
Christine Craggs-Hinton

Chronic Fatigue Syndrome: What you need to know about CFS/ME
Dr Megan A. Arroll

The Chronic Pain Diet Book
Neville Shone

Cider Vinegar
Margaret Hills

Coeliac Disease: What you need to know
Alex Gazzola

Coping Successfully with Chronic Illness: Your healing plan
Neville Shone

Coping Successfully with Hiatus Hernia
Dr Tom Smith

Coping Successfully with Pain
Neville Shone

Coping Successfully with Panic Attacks
Shirley Trickett

Coping Successfully with Prostate Cancer
Dr Tom Smith

Coping Successfully with Shyness
Margaret Oakes, Professor Robert Bor and Dr Carina Eriksen

Coping Successfully with Ulcerative Colitis
Peter Cartwright

Coping Successfully with Varicose Veins
Christine Craggs-Hinton

Coping Successfully with Your Irritable Bowel
Rosemary Nicol

Coping with a Mental Health Crisis: Seven steps to healing
Catherine G. Lucas

Coping with Asthma in Adults
Mark Greener

Coping with Blushing
Professor Robert J. Edelmann

Coping with Bronchitis and Emphysema
Dr Tom Smith

Coping with Chemotherapy
Dr Terry Priestman

Coping with Coeliac Disease: Strategies to change your diet and life
Karen Brody

Coping with Difficult Families
Dr Jane McGregor and Tim McGregor

Coping with Diverticulitis
Peter Cartwright

Coping with Dyspraxia
Jill Eckersley

Coping with Early-onset Dementia
Jill Eckersley

Coping with Endometriosis
Jill Eckersley and Dr Zara Aziz

Coping with Epilepsy
Dr Pamela Crawford and Fiona Marshall

Coping with Gout
Christine Craggs-Hinton

Coping with Guilt
Dr Windy Dryden

Coping with Headaches and Migraine
Alison Frith

Coping with Heartburn and Reflux
Dr Tom Smith

Overcoming Common Problems

Dr Dawn's Guide to Your Baby's First Year

DR DAWN HARPER

sheldon **PRESS**
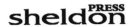

First published in Great Britain in 2016

Sheldon Press
36 Causton Street
London SW1P 4ST
www.sheldonpress.co.uk

Copyright © Dr Dawn Harper 2016

British Library Cataloguing-in-Publication Data
A catalogue record for this book is available from the British Library

ISBN 978–1–84709–392–9
eBook ISBN 978–1–84709–397–4

Typeset by Fakenham Prepress Solutions, Fakenham, Norfolk NR21 8NN
First printed in Great Britain by Ashford Colour Press
Subsequently digitally reprinted in Great Britain

eBook by Fakenham Prepress Solutions, Fakenham, Norfolk NR21 8NN

Produced on paper from sustainable forests

To my firstborn son, Charlie.
Thank you for all the special firsts

Contents

Introduction

My first baby was a big baby, 9 pounds 5 ounces big to be precise, and as a result he was born by emergency caesarean section. I had planned to have a hospital delivery and come straight home but, of course, the operation took that decision out of my hands and in retrospect I'm glad it did. In the last few weeks of my pregnancy members of my family and friends who already had children kept asking me if I was sure, telling me that I would be tired and that 'having your first baby is a big deal you know'. I remember thinking, 'Just how big a deal can this be?' I had after all looked after hundreds of babies in special care baby units. I had set up drips, done lumbar punctures, ventilated premature babies and could calculate the dose of any drug to the nearest 0.1 of a gram for virtually any condition. Just how hard was it going to be to change a nappy and feed my beautiful new baby?

What my friends and family knew then, and what I know now, is that, just like any other first-time mum, I was about to be launched into parenthood without a handbook, and while it may not necessarily be difficult it was, without doubt, totally and utterly daunting.

I remember a nurse opening the door to my room the morning after I had had my son and asking me if I would like her to help me bath my baby. I, of course, accepted only to see matron swing in to the room to explain that I was a GP and I would know what to do. I assured her I absolutely didn't and I would really appreciate her guidance. I watched as she tucked my son into the crook of her left arm and ran water into a plastic baby bath while testing the temperature with her right elbow. All I could think was that I would *never* be able to do that. I would be too scared of dropping my baby. That was the beginning of many firsts.

I remember coming home and wondering if I would ever be able to get out of the house before midday again! How difficult can it be to wash and dress a baby and myself I kept asking? The answer, of course, was quite difficult when you are on a steep learning curve.

My first child is 21 years old now but my memories of his first year are very strong. There is nothing quite so wonderful as watching your baby grow and develop. I also know that with every development come new anxieties and new questions, which is why I wanted to write this book. I hope it will help you enjoy your baby and his or her first year to the full.

1

Let's start with you

The first few weeks after your baby is born are likely to keep your postman busy with cards and presents from well-wishers. I remember our cottage looked like a small branch of a baby clothing store – we had so many baby clothes! Some friends (mainly those who had had children themselves) thought ahead and bought larger sizes but one present in particular stands out in my mind and that was a box of beautiful toiletries from a fellow GP. The card simply read 'Congratulations! ... Don't forget about you'.

As a doctor and mother of three, my colleague knew how easy it is to neglect yourself when a new baby arrives. It is normal to feel tired, and only a very tiny number of women slip straight back into their favourite jeans, but you don't need to be a bag lady either. Taking care of yourself will help you feel more feminine and give you confidence in your body.

It is likely to take several weeks for you to regain your pre-pregnancy figure and while you don't want to spend a lot of money on clothes that you don't intend to wear for long it is worth investing in a few new things. Your maternity clothes will probably be too big but there is nothing worse than squeezing yourself into uncomfortably tight waistbands for making you feel like two tonne Tessie. Don't forget you have carried your baby for nine months and probably worked hard during labour – you deserve a treat.

A well-fitted maternity bra is a must and every woman feels more feminine in new pants. If you are still losing lochia, choose a darker colour that won't show the stains so readily. You may need a new pair of jeans and if you really can't face needing a larger size then cut the label out and forget about it – no one else knows what size you are wearing and you will look and feel better in clothes that fit. Leggings are cheap and comfortable, and with a few pretty accessories can look stylish. You can afford to be a little more extravagant when it comes to tops as they will stay in your wardrobe for longer.

1

If you are breastfeeding, remember you will need to choose your style to allow for this and dark colours or patterns make it less obvious if you leak milk.

Simple things like painting your toenails (after all you can actually reach them now!) will make you feel more attractive and, while you probably won't have the time or the inclination for a complete makeover, lipstick and a drop of perfume will mean you feel like a woman as well as a mum.

Sex is off the agenda for most women in the early days but that doesn't mean you shouldn't enjoy some intimacy with your partner. The more attractive you feel the more confident you will be in your own body, so it's worth taking a little bit of time out when you can to look after yourself.

Dr Dawn's top tips for having some 'me time'

- *Make the most of when your baby is sleeping* There is nothing wrong with soaking in a bubble bath, shaving your legs and doing your hair at two in the afternoon if that's when the opportunity arises and it will make you feel so much better about yourself.
- *If you are breastfeeding, try to express early on* Having a supply of breast milk to hand means that someone else can give the occasional feed meaning you and your partner can take the opportunity to be a couple again even if it is only for an hour or two.
- *Accept offers of help* Friends and family really do want to help and if they offer to sit with your baby while you pop round to see a friend or nip to the shops say 'Yes, please!' It's normal to feel that no one else can look after your baby as well as you but you are only human and the truth is you will be an even better mum if you can take a few minutes out here and there, so don't feel guilty. Do it in the full knowledge that when you get back, you will be refreshed and able to give even more of yourself.

2

Feeding and weaning

Breastfeeding

During your pregnancy you will have noticed changes in your breasts as they prepare for you to breastfeed your baby. There is no doubt that breast milk is the best food for your new arrival, but breastfeeding can take some working at. A bit like learning to ride a bike, it comes more naturally to some than others. Of course whether or not you breastfeed is entirely a personal choice and no one should be made to feel guilty about how they decide to feed their baby. My own view is that there are so many benefits to both mother and baby that breastfeeding is well worth a try. I hope that this chapter will answer any concerns you may have and give you the tips you need to give you the best chance to breastfeed your baby happily.

The benefits of breastfeeding

Benefits to your baby

Breast milk is the perfect food for a newborn baby, containing just the right balance of protein, carbohydrate and fat to allow your baby to thrive, but it's not just nutrients that your baby will get from breast milk. Breastfed babies also receive antibodies to protect them from illnesses such as gastroenteritis and chest and ear infections. The balance of breast milk is so good that it is almost impossible to overfeed a breastfed baby so they won't be overweight, and breast milk is more easily digested than formula, meaning that breastfed babies don't get constipated. The stools they pass are also free of bacteria so they are less smelly, and the baby is less likely to develop nappy rash.

Did you know?

Breastfed babies are:

- five times less likely to be admitted to hospital with diarrhoea and vomiting as a baby;
- less prone to severe respiratory infections;
- at lower risk of ear and urinary tract infections;
- more likely to score higher on tests of neurological development;
- less likely to develop allergies later in life;
- less likely to develop insulin-dependent diabetes as a child;
- less prone to being overweight or having higher blood pressure as children.

Benefits to you

The great thing about breastfeeding is that, once your milk has 'come in', you always have a supply of sterilized milk at the correct temperature and, of course, it's free but there are other less obvious benefits. Mothers who breastfeed are less likely to develop breast cancer later in life and, a subject close to most women's hearts, breastfeeding mums usually find it easier to get their figure back in shape. During pregnancy we all gain extra weight in the form of fat stores laid down in preparation for breastfeeding. When I was breastfeeding, I used to joke that my babies were my own personal liposuction machines and research has shown that in many ways they are! Women who breastfeed find their pelvis and waistline return to normal more quickly. In fact, breastfeeding uses around 500 calories a day.

How is breast milk produced?

In order to understand how breast milk is produced, we need to know a bit about the anatomy of the breast which is in fact made up of 15 to 20 lobes (Figure 1). In each lobe are clusters of cells responsible for producing and storing breast milk. Milk ducts link the lobes to sinuses below the areola (the dark area around your nipple) and these sinuses then release milk through 15 to 20 openings in the nipple (Figure 2). The cells responsible for producing milk are deep in the breast tissue below the more

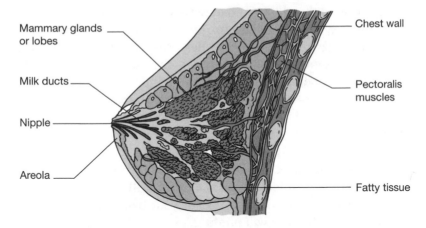

Figure 1 Anatomy of the breast

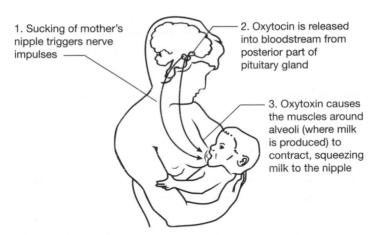

Figure 2 Milk production

superficial fatty tissue so how much milk you can produce has nothing to do with the size of your breasts. Even very small-chested women are perfectly capable of producing plenty of milk for their babies.

The release of breast milk is controlled by a complex inter-action of nerve impulses and hormones. As a baby sucks, the nerve endings around the nipple send messages to the brain to release two hormones, oxytocin and prolactin. Oxytocin, also called the cuddle hormone, triggers the let-down reflex. This means the cells deep in the breast squeeze milk up through the ducts. Lots of women experience a tingling sensation in the nipple as this happens. A few find it more intense and briefly uncomfortable and some don't actually feel it at all, but this doesn't mean it isn't happening. The let-down reflex is so sensitive in some new mums that simply the sound of their baby crying is enough to trigger it.

The second hormone, prolactin, is responsible for stimulating the production of more milk and this is nature's brilliant way of making sure you always have enough milk for your baby. The more he or she sucks, the more you will produce.

Changes to your breast milk

Unlike formula milk, which is always the same, breast milk changes its composition slightly both during an individual feed and over the weeks that you feed, meaning that your baby has his or her own tailor made diet, fine tuned specifically for baby's needs. There are four stages of milk production – colostrum, transitional milk, foremilk and hindmilk.

- *Colostrum* This is the first milk your breast produces and it looks richer and more yellow than other milk. You will only produce 3 or 4 teaspoons a day, but it is packed with antibodies and a substance called lactoferrin, which has natural antibiotic activity and has more protein than mature breast milk. In an ideal world, I like to see mums breastfeed for six months but even if you don't want to breastfeed long term, it is well worth considering giving your baby the benefit of colostrum, which is only produced for the first couple of days, as it will help boost your baby's immune system and works as a laxative to clear the meconium (the first dark green stools) from your baby's bowels.
- *Transitional milk* After two or three days, the colostrum is replaced by transitional milk and this is what people mean when they refer to your milk 'coming in'. Transitional milk is thinner than colostrum and therefore gives the impression that it is

flowing more easily. After a couple of weeks, your breastfeeding will be well-established and your breasts will produce mature milk, which is made up of foremilk and hindmilk.

- *Foremilk* Foremilk is thin and watery. It may even have a blueish tinge to it and it is designed to quench your baby's thirst before his or her meal. Baby's very own aperitif!
- *Hindmilk* The hindmilk is your baby's starter, main and pudding. It is thicker than foremilk and contains all the protein, fat and nutrients he or she needs to develop.

Once breastfeeding is established, your breasts will produce anything up to a litre of milk a day, which is plenty for your growing baby.

When the milk comes in

The first few days of feeding your new baby can be quite an anxious time for new mums so here are a few of the common questions I am asked.

How will I know when my milk comes in?

For the first couple of days you will produce just 3–4 teaspoons a day of a rich milk called colostrum. On day two or three you will notice the milk looks clearer and is more plentiful. This is your milk coming in.

What if I don't feel a let-down reflex?

A let-down reflex is a tingling sensation around your nipple which some women feel as their baby begins to suckle. Some even feel it when their baby cries but others don't notice it at all. It doesn't matter – you will still produce enough milk.

Is it normal to have period pain when breastfeeding?

Yes. The hormone that triggers the let-down reflex also makes your uterus contract causing what is known as after pains. This is normal and is more common in women who have had children before.

Getting started

Ideally, you should make the decision about whether or not to breastfeed before your baby is born so that you can prepare. If you have flat or inverted nipples you may find it useful to encourage the nipple out with a niplette during pregnancy (see FAQs).

I think it is well worth investing in a couple of well-fitted maternity bras, the best you can afford as they will make life easier and more comfortable, and a supply of breast pads. If you are going to breastfeed, your breasts will leak from time to time and you can bet your bottom dollar it will happen just when you don't want it to. Breast pads certainly saved me from a few embarrassing moments! While we are on the subject, you may want to think about your wardrobe too. Loose-fitting T-shirts and sweatshirts are easier to feed from discreetly if you are in company than buttoned shirts, and dark colours will be more forgiving when it comes to leaking milk.

Latching on and releasing the nipple

Before you start feeding, make sure that you are comfortable and that your baby is well supported. Remember you could be there for at least 20 minutes. If you position yourself so that your nipple is level with your baby's nose, baby will smell your milk and open his or her mouth. Gently stroking baby's cheek will trigger a reflex called the 'rooting reflex', that will encourage your baby to turn toward your breast. Now baby is in the best position to 'latch on' and by that we mean take as much of the breast as possible into his or her mouth. Ideally, baby should have the nipple and most of the areola (the dark area of skin around the nipple) in his or her mouth and the bottom lip should be curled back. A baby's suck is quite vigorous and if baby takes just the nipple into his or her mouth, it won't be long before you feel sore.

When you watch your baby feeding, you will see baby's jaw muscles working in a rhythm as far back as the angle of the jaw. If baby's cheeks are caving in, he or she is not latched on properly so gently place your little finger into the corner of baby's mouth to release baby and try again.

Your baby will let you know when he or she has had enough by simply letting the breast fall from the mouth, but if baby falls asleep on the breast you can release him or her by placing your little finger in the corner of the mouth.

Positions for breastfeeding

There are no hard and fast rules here. The bottom line is that both you and your baby must be comfortable. My mother gave me a nursing chair when my first child was born. I remember thinking it was an extravagance but it turned out to be such an asset. It had a low seat and high back, which gave me great support and it is still one of the most popular chairs in my lounge! Experiment with different seats in your home and you will soon find what works best for you and remember, this is not a time to be rushed.

Cradle hold Probably the most popular (Figure 3) but it's not the only option and if you are struggling with breastfeeding it's worth trying some of the alternatives.

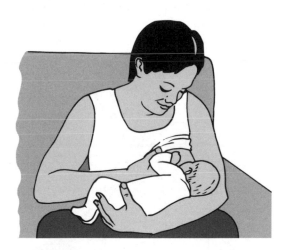

Figure 3 Cradle hold

Cross cradle hold This position allows you to cuddle your baby while feeding. Using a pillow to support your arms as you hold your baby will prevent your arms from tiring (Figure 4 overleaf).

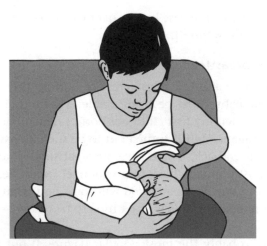

Figure 4 Cross cradle hold

Football hold This position frees your hands up so if you are having difficulty getting your baby to latch on, one hand can manoeuvre the breast towards your baby's mouth while the other supports his or her head (Figure 5).

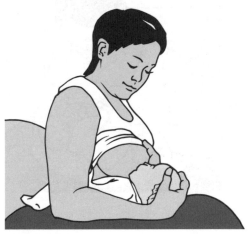

Figure 5 Football hold

Side lying position Again, this allows your hands freedom to help out if you have issues with latching on and it's a great position for mums who have had a caesarean section and find it uncomfortable to have their baby lying on the tummy (Figure 6). Do make sure that you don't fall asleep while feeding and smother your baby.

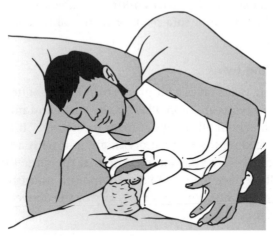

Figure 6 Side lying position

Saddle hold Again, a great one if your tummy is a bit tender after a caesarean section and one I enjoyed during night feeds but, again, make sure that you don't fall asleep and smother your baby. You may need to lie a small baby on a pillow so that baby can reach your breast (Figure 7). Your baby needs to have good head control for this one, but it's a good one for older babies still breastfeeding.

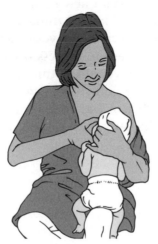

Figure 7 Saddle hold

Whatever positions work for you, remember, feeding is a time to relax and enjoy that special bond with your baby and it needn't be a time to exclude the other children. I have lovely memories of being cuddled up on a sofa reading to my older children as I fed my youngest.

Breastfeeding twins

Breastfeeding twins takes a bit more effort but it is effort well worth making since twins are more likely to be small and may have come early so will benefit all the more from breast milk. It may be easier to start by feeding the twins individually but with a bit of help, it won't be long before you can feed them at the same time and your breasts will produce plenty to keep them both nourished. With the exception of the side lying position, any of the above positions can be adapted for twins.

Breastfeeding premature babies

Premature babies are more likely to spend time in a special care baby unit (SCBU) and babies born very early may not have an established sucking reflex so may need to be fed by a tube through the nose into the stomach. The problem is, premature babies are the most vulnerable when it comes to infections and other problems so they, more than any other baby, need the protection of breast milk. It's a dilemma for new mums and one that I had with two of my three children. The first thing to do is to make sure that all the doctors and nurses caring for your baby know that you want to breastfeed. You will need to express the milk and the staff will then be able to give it to your baby through a tube until he or she is strong enough to feed normally. There's no doubt that a baby's suckle is the most efficient way of getting milk out of the breast and expressing in the early days can be difficult but it is worth persevering.

Dr Dawn's top tips on maintaining a good milk supply

- *Rest*! Most of your milk is produced in the morning when you are rested. If you are rushing around making cups of tea and cake for every well wisher, you could find they are well fed and watered but your baby isn't.
- Accept offers of help. People really do want to support you. If you are breastfeeding, they can't necessarily feed your baby but they can provide a meal for the rest of the family or entertain older children.
- Drink plenty – you will need at least 3 litres of fluid a day to keep up a good milk supply.
- Eat a well-balanced diet rich in protein and avoid too many complex carbohydrates such as cakes and biscuits.
- Relax – taking some time out each day for relaxation will improve your milk supply.
- If you have to be away from your baby for a feed, find the time to express some milk so that you keep the supply going.

FAQs

How often should I feed?

I have never been a subscriber to the idea that your baby should be fed by the clock. Babies need to feed frequently and breastfed babies may need more feeds than bottle-fed babies because they digest their milk more quickly. Newborn babies may feed ten times a day but by one month it is normal for a baby to feed every three hours or so, and by two or three months it will be more like every four hours. These numbers are just a rough guide though and as a mum you will tune into your own baby's needs. Try not to get too hung up on times. If your baby seems hungry, offer a feed – baby will soon let you know if that's what he or she wants!

In general, most babies sleep through the night at three or four months old but that isn't always the case. My first son had definitely not read the right baby books and was nearly a year old before I had my first undisturbed night!

How long should I leave my baby on each breast?

As a rough guide, your baby will have taken 80 per cent of his or her feed in the first five minutes and will have finished five minutes later, so ten minutes on each breast should be about right but some babies feed more quickly than others and some enjoy continuing to suckle after they have finished feeding. As long as you are comfortable, there is no reason why you shouldn't allow this. It is important that your baby empties one breast before being offered the other so that you can be sure that he or she is getting the nutrient-rich hindmilk. If baby then doesn't want the second breast, this isn't a problem, just remember to offer baby the unused side first for the next feed.

I have inverted nipples, will I be able to breastfeed?

Inverted nipples are much more common than most people realize – about one in ten women have flat or inverted nipples and the good news is, most of them manage to breastfeed perfectly well. You may find it helpful to use a niplette during pregnancy. This is a small device that looks like a thimble and can be placed over the nipple. You then apply some gentle suction using a syringe attached to the other end to draw the nipple out. You can also use it in the first few days after delivery before each feed. When your milk comes in fully, your breasts will become more engorged and it won't work but by that stage your baby will probably have learned how to latch on. Some of my patients have found using a breast pump, or expressing a little milk by hand before feeds helps if you still have problems.

What if my breasts feel engorged and tender?

It is normal for breasts to feel tense and swollen particularly as your milk starts to come in properly, usually a few days after your baby is born. It can take a day or two for your milk supply to settle down and for your body to adapt to produce the right amount of milk for your baby. You will feel more comfortable if you feed your baby little and often to prevent the milk supply from building up. Engorged breasts can make it difficult for your baby to latch on though and if this is the case, simply express a little milk by hand before the start of each feed.

Can I mix breastfeeding and bottle-feeding?

If you are breastfeeding successfully, it is best for your baby if they receive all their feeds as breast milk but that's not to say that some of them couldn't be from a bottle as expressed milk. Some babies who are used to breastfeeding object to a plastic teat and refuse bottle-feeds but with a bit of perseverance you should succeed. Sometimes a baby will take milk from a bottle better if you are not around.

When you are ready to wean your baby from the breast then substituting occasional feeds with formula feeds from a bottle is an excellent way to reduce your milk supply slowly and prevent your breasts becoming engorged.

Is it safe to take medication when I am breastfeeding?

Some medicines are passed on in breast milk and some aren't, but it's safest to assume that anything you take could be passed on to your baby so always check with your GP or pharmacist before taking any prescription or over-the-counter medicines. If you are taking regular medication and are planning to breastfeed, make sure you discuss this with your GP during your pregnancy. It may be that you will need to swap to an alternative treatment while you breastfeed so you will need to think ahead.

Are there any medical reasons not to breastfeed?

Breast milk as I have said is full of a natural balance of nutrients but it may not contain enough vitamin D, which is why all breast-feeding mothers are advised to take vitamin D supplements in the UK. If you are HIV positive, it is possible for the virus to be spread through breast milk and your GP will advise on whether you and your baby should be taking anti-retroviral medicines while you breastfeed. There are some other infections that may mean your GP suggests you suspend breastfeeding for a short period of time (usually around 48 hours). These include gonorrhoea, haemo-philus, group B streptococcus, staphylococcus and Lyme disease.

Will my breasts sag if I breastfeed?

No. Contrary to popular belief, there is no correlation between breastfeeding and saggy boobs.

Can I breastfeed if I have had breast surgery?

Almost certainly, yes. If you have had surgery around the nipple, there could have been damage to some of the ducts or nerve endings that may make it a little more difficult to establish breast-feeding but I have lots of patients who have had breast surgery including implants, who have breastfed successfully.

Common problems with breastfeeding

Cracked nipples

Nipples can become sore when breastfeeding, particularly if you have fair skin or if your baby doesn't always latch on properly. You can minimize the risks of them developing into cracked nipples by positioning your baby properly to feed (see Latching on and releasing the nipple) and ensuring that your nipple is dry before putting your bra back on. Wearing absorbent breast pads between feeds also helps. Silicone shields available from chemists fit over the nipple and allow the baby to suck through a small teat at the front, but if you need to use these, remember to sterilize them between feeds. If the nipple actually cracks, you will probably need to express milk from that side but continue to feed normally from the other. It's natural and right to want to keep your breasts clean when you are breastfeeding but you only need to use water and maybe some baby lotion. Don't use soap as this tends to dry the skin and can make you more prone to cracked nipples.

Thrush

Thrush is a fungal infection that can spread from your baby's mouth to your breast making it sore and itchy. The good news is that it is easy to treat and you shouldn't need to stop breastfeeding. You can reduce your risk of thrush by taking a daily probiotic, keeping your nipples dry and avoiding using any perfumed products, including soap, on your breasts.

Blocked milk ducts

If a milk duct becomes blocked, you will notice a hard red patch usually in the outside of the breast. It is important to help that duct to drain by feeding from that breast first so that it is fully emptied, and expressing milk if necessary. Wearing a properly fitted feeding bra and altering feeding positions throughout the day should help prevent this problem recurring.

Mastitis

Mastitis is miserable. It makes you feel hot and fluey and the breast becomes red and painful, but it is easily treated with antibiotics and your GP will make sure that the antibiotics you are prescribed are safe for your baby so you will be able to continue feeding. Lying in a warm bath with hot flannels on the affected breast is soothing and gently massaging the breast toward the nipple will encourage the milk to flow. Wherever possible, even if it is a bit sore, it is best to try to continue feeding to avoid any further engorgement.

Contraception and breastfeeding

Your fertility is reduced while you are breastfeeding, but not enough for you to be able to rely on it as a form of contraception! Your postnatal check is a good time to chat to your GP about the many contraceptive options available to you but avoid the combined contraceptive pill while you are breastfeeding as it can interfere with your milk supply.

Expressing milk

There are a number of scenarios where you may want to express some milk. Maybe your breasts are becoming engorged or you may want to leave a supply of your milk for someone else to give if you have to be away from your baby for a while. You can express by hand into a sterile container or there are a variety of pumps available. Which you use is down to personal preference but it is essential that you make sure your hands are clean and all equipment is sterilized before you start. Expressed milk will store in a fridge for up to 48 hours and can be kept in the freezer for anything up to six months.

Expressing by hand

Find a comfortable position where you can position your breast over the collecting container without having to bend awkwardly. Hold your breast in both hands and gently squeeze the outer part of your breast between your fingers and thumbs. Repeat this movement several times and then move your hand forward doing the same thing. This stimulates the milk forward from the deeper part of the breast. This will take a few seconds and then you can gently squeeze around the areola to produce your milk.

Expressing using a pump

There are lots of different designs of pump and you will need to get familiar with your chosen brand. You will have a funnel-shaped opening that needs to be placed over the nipple. Just as a baby needs to latch on properly it is important to cover as much of the areola as possible and ensure you have a good seal.

Bottle-feeding

If you decide you want to bottle-feed your baby, you will need to think ahead and make sure you have all the equipment at home. You will need bottles, teats, sterilizing equipment and infant formula. Formula milk can be bought in cartons, which have been heat-treated so they are sterilized and safe to use at any time before the sell-by date. Once opened the carton should be stored in a fridge and used within 24 hours. This is a more expensive option and most bottle-fed babies will be fed primarily with infant formula powdered milk, which can be made up according to the instructions. Always follow the instructions exactly to the letter. Don't be tempted to add extra powder or less unless specifically advised to do so by your GP or health visitor. Use cooled, boiled tap water to make up the bottles. The instructions will say how many scoops of powder to add – use a clean knife to level off each scoop so that you know the amounts are correct. Give the bottle a good shake to ensure the contents are well mixed and always test the temperature by tipping a little milk on to the inside of your own wrist. It should feel warm not hot.

Just like breastfeeding, make sure you and your baby are comfortable. When you are bottle-feeding you will need to tip the bottle at an angle so that the teat is full of milk to avoid allowing your baby to gulp air rather than milk.

It is best to make up each feed as it is needed but there will inevitably be times when you need to prepare in advance, if you are going out for the day for example or if your baby goes to childcare. In these instances, it is fine to store pre-prepared formula for up to 12 hours in a fridge or for 4 hours in a cool bag. You will need to warm the milk before offering it to your baby. You can do this by standing it in a bowl of warm water for 15 minutes or if you need to do this frequently, you can buy electric bottle warmers. I'm not a fan of using microwaves to warm infant formula as they can heat unevenly and you could risk having hot pockets of milk in the bottle.

Most babies will thrive on formula made from cow's milk but if your GP suspects a cow's milk allergy he or she may suggest you try a hydrolysed protein infant formula. There are also soya-based and goat's milk infant formulae but babies who are allergic to cow's milk may also be allergic to these.

Sterilizing bottles

Sterilizing your bottles is vital for your baby's health. Whether you are using expressed milk or formula milk, all the bottles and teats should be cleaned properly after every feed. Clean the bottle and teat in hot soapy water using a bottle brush, which should be reserved for this purpose, and then rinse thoroughly in cold water. There are several different ways of sterilizing your equipment.

- *Boiling* Put all the items in a large pan, making sure that they are all completely immersed in water. Bring the pan to the boil and leave the items in the boiling water for ten minutes.
- *Cold water sterilizing* You can buy sterilizing solution. Simply immerse the bottles and teats for 30 minutes, after which time they will be sterilized. Remember to change the sterilizing solution every 24 hours.
- *Microwave* Wash the bottles and half fill them with water, then stand them upright and microwave for about one minute and a half. Teats can be sterilized by putting them in a bowl covered with water and placing them in the microwave with the bottles.

- *Electric sterilizer* You need to place bottles and teats facing downwards in an electric sterilizer and follow the manufacturer's instructions, as there are several different types that you can buy.

If you are not going to use the bottles immediately after sterilizing them, put the teat and lid firmly in place to keep them clean.

Burping your baby

Babies vary hugely. My first was a great guzzler and needed lots of burping, while his sister was the exact opposite. Breastfed babies tend to need less burping than bottle-fed babies simply because they swallow less air while feeding. Your baby will tell you if he or she needs burping. The baby that falls asleep after a feed and is contented should be left to do so. There is no need to burp baby. But if your baby looks uncomfortable and is fidgety, try burping. You can do this by placing baby against your chest, supporting his or her upper back and head with one hand and gently rubbing or patting the middle of baby's back with the other. Or you can sit baby on your lap facing away from you and supporting the chest or tummy with one hand you can rub or pat with the other, or simply lie baby face down on your lap and, keeping baby's head slightly up with one hand, you can wind baby with the other. If your baby is struggling with wind, talk to your health visitor about massage techniques that she can teach you.

Weaning

The NHS recommends that we start solid foods at around six months of age. Babies are very different and some may be ready earlier, although we don't recommend weaning on to solids before four months. If you do start solids before six months, avoid wheat, gluten, nuts, seeds, liver, cow's milk, fish, shellfish and unpasteurized cheeses as these can trigger allergies in very young infants. In the early days you and your baby can simply experiment with different foods. Your baby will still be getting most of his or her nutrition from formula or breast milk and it can be some time before you get into a routine of three meals a day. For a baby to be able to start eating solid foods, he or she must be able to sit up, co-ordinate his or her eyes and hands and to be able to chew and swallow. If your baby was born prematurely, it may take longer for these skills to develop but your health visitor and doctors will advise you.

When you start solids it is important that you stay close to your baby. Don't leave them in a high chair with a plate of finger food in case they start choking. And in the beginning remember this is as much about exploring and having fun as it is about nutrition.

The first foods to try will include things like cooked mashed potato, carrot or parsnip or fruit like banana, apple or pear. Or you may like to try baby rice or baby cereal mixed with your baby's milk. Breast or formula milk will continue to be the main drink but you can start to offer sips of water from a beaker anytime from six months.

As soon as your baby has mastered the art of solids you can start to explore other foods. People often worry about introducing eggs and meat but well-cooked meat and mashed hard-boiled eggs are fine at this stage. It is also fine to use cow's milk to mix food at this stage but babies should not be given cow's milk to drink until 12 months old. It is important that you keep things as healthy as possible at this stage. You don't want your little one to develop a taste for salty or sugary foods so don't add any to their food. There is also some evidence that if you leave the food with some texture and distinct flavours at around eight to nine months then your baby is less likely to be a faddy eater later in life so don't mush your meal into a pulp; let your baby taste meat and vegetables individually and with a bit of texture. All babies from six months to five years should be given vitamin drops containing vitamins A, C and D.

3

Bathing and hygiene

It's important that your baby is kept clean but contrary to popular belief it isn't essential for your baby to have a bath every day. When mine were little bath time was part of bedtime and that worked for me but as long as your baby is having a bath two to three times a week and being 'topped and tailed' on the other days, baby will be fine.

What is topping and tailing?

To top and tail your baby, place baby on a changing mat without any clothes or a nappy on and wrap baby in a soft warm towel. You will need a bowl of warm water and clean cotton wool. Using a different piece for each eye, dip the cotton wool in the water and squeeze the excess water out. Then use the cotton wool to wipe each eye clean. Using fresh cotton wool wipe around his or her ears but not in them and don't ever be tempted to use cotton wool buds in a baby's ear. The skin lining the ear canal is very delicate and easily damaged. Wash the rest of your baby's face in the same way taking care to pay attention to under the chin and then dry in the towel. 'Tailing' involves doing the same thing around the bottom and the skin creases around the genital area.

Preparing to bath your baby

It's a good idea to get everything ready before you start bath time and make sure the room is a comfortable temperature. Fill the baby bath with about 20–25 centimetres of water. Start with cold water and then add the hot, mix well and always check the temperature by dipping your elbow in the water. The water should feel the same as your body temperature. You can gently lower your baby into the water while supporting the head and upper neck and then gently swish the water around baby. There is no need to add bubble baths

23

to the water and you can wash your baby's hair with plain water too. It is best not to use any other products at all in the first month (longer in premature babies). After that if you want to use a bubble bath choose one that is pH balanced and has minimal colouring or perfume as these can sensitize such delicate skin. And only use them two or three times a week. You shouldn't need to use any shampoo for the first year of your baby's life. After a bath, make sure you dry your baby properly taking care not to miss any skin creases but be gentle – a baby's skin is very delicate.

Cutting your baby's nails

You would be amazed how long some newborn babies' nails are! It is important that they are cut so that your baby can't scratch him- or herself. You can buy special baby clippers or safety scissors from your pharmacist to do this.

When should I start brushing my baby's teeth?

You can start brushing your baby's teeth as soon as they appear, which is usually at around six months. It is important to be very gentle and make the whole experience pleasurable. Use a soft baby toothbrush and a tiny smear of fluoride toothpaste. It is probably easiest to sit small babies on your lap with their back to you and using gentle circular movements, clean the teeth. It's good to get into the habit of doing this twice a day.

4

Sleeping

When it comes to sleeping, it's important to remember that, just like adults, babies are all individuals and some will need more sleep than others. My first son seemed to barely sleep at all and when his sister came along 18 months later I remember waking in a blind panic thinking the worst when I realized I had slept through the night, but there she was sleeping peacefully in her cot beside me. She was just very different from her brother and still is! The important thing is to try to go with the flow in the early days. All babies will eventually find a routine, but if you try to be too rigid about sleep and feeding you are more likely to cause yourself more stress and your baby will pick up on that.

If your baby is sleeping during the day, take advantage of the opportunity to get a bit of rest yourself. I'm not a fan of taking daytime catnaps as a rule, but napping when you are a new mum is one great big exception! If your baby is waking several times in the night and you are exhausted, you could try waking baby just before you go to bed for a feed so that hopefully baby will sleep a bit longer before needing another one. If you are breastfeeding and exhausted, try expressing some milk so that maybe your partner could do one of the night feeds at weekends.

The first three months can feel like everything is upside down, but after three months you might be able to start introducing more of a routine. This was where I found bath time really useful. I would bath my babies quietly. (When they got older bath time became more raucous and, while still part of the routine, I found I had to work harder at winding them down after a load of giggles and fun in the bath!) After a bath, change your baby into night clothes and feed baby, perhaps while you sing or you play some music in the background. All sounds so easy I know and it doesn't always go to plan, but if you persevere your baby should soon learn that this is all part of going to bed and ideally you should be able to leave your baby contented even if not asleep. If you always wait until your baby has dozed off, you could be creating a rod for your own back as baby will soon learn that he or she can get you to stay for longer.

How do I know if my baby is getting enough sleep?

The wonderful thing about babies is that they can sleep through pretty much anything! They will get enough sleep and, even if the whole street pop in and it gets rather noisy, a tired baby will sleep through it.

As a rough guide most newborn babies will spend more time asleep than they do awake and may sleep as much as 18 hours a day. At about three months some babies will sleep eight hours through the night, but not all will. Breast milk is more easily digested than formula milk so breastfed babies may be more prone to waking for a night feed. By about four months most babies will spend twice as much time asleep at night as they do during the day. From six months they may sleep for up to 12 hours at night.

Where should my baby sleep at night?

I had all three of my children in the same room as me for the first six months. It did mean that I heard every noise and probably had more disturbed nights but that is what is recommended by the NHS. It is best to have them in a cot next to you and not in your bed with you, as you risk them overheating with your body heat and your bedclothes.

What is the best temperature for a baby's bedroom?

Babies cannot control their body temperature in the same way as adults do so it is important that we keep their environment at a steady temperature. The ideal temperature for a baby's bedroom is 16–20 degrees centigrade. You can check that with a simple room thermometer.

What position should my baby sleep in?

It is important that babies are put to sleep on their backs. This is to reduce the risk of cot death (see below). We don't really know why this position is safer, but there are a number of theories. One is that a baby sleeping on its front may be breathing the same air, another is that they could suffocate in a soft mattress, which is why we advise that a baby's mattress should be firm and horizontal. Once a baby can turn over independently baby may well roll on to his or her front. There is no need to move the baby back.

Cot death

Cot death, also known as sudden infant death syndrome (SIDS), is every parent's worst nightmare, but thankfully it is rare – affecting about 1 in 3,000 babies. That's about 270 babies a year in the UK. It occurs most commonly in young babies aged between two and four months. By the time a baby is able to roll over (usually around five months) the risks start to fall and cot death is rare over the age of one year.

What can I do to reduce the risk of cot death?

If you or your partner smoke, your baby is at increased risk of cot death, so if you can't give up for each other, this is a really good incentive to try now. Your GP will be able to advise you about local smoking cessation clinics and we know your chances of success at quitting are greater if you do it with help. Other things you should do include:

- breastfeed if you can – breastfed babies have a reduced risk of cot death;
- always put your baby to sleep on his or her back;
- avoid pillows or lots of soft toys in baby's bed;
- do not sleep with your baby in your bed or on a sofa;
- keep the room at an optimum temperature of 16–20 degrees;
- only cover your baby up to the shoulders with sheets rather than duvets;
- offer a dummy at night. We don't know why this works but babies offered a dummy to go to sleep at night have a reduced incidence of cot death.

5

Travelling with your baby

In the early days you are unlikely to feel like travelling anywhere! As I said in the introduction of this book, when I brought my first child home from hospital it took me the entire morning just to get him and myself washed and dressed. But, as you start to settle into your routine, you will want to take your baby out and about to meet people and give you both different experiences. Whether you are planning a trip abroad or a shopping trip to your local town, travelling with a baby takes some planning.

The first thing you need to do is to pack appropriately. If it's a quick outing for a coffee with another mum you obviously need less than for a foreign holiday, but it is worth taking slightly more than you need to allow for any unexpected delays. I used to laugh that the smaller my children were, the more paraphernalia I needed to take with me, which is of course true, but the flip side is that small babies are easily transportable and won't object to your choice of destination!

Dr Dawn's checklist for what to pack

Knowing that you have all that you are likely to need will take the stress out of travelling. This is my 'must have' list:

- baby bag, complete with changing mat, spare nappies, nappy sacks and wipes
- pushchair or sling
- travel cot, if staying overnight
- feeding equipment
- sterilizing equipment.

Travelling by car

Your baby will need to be strapped into a car seat that is appropriate for baby's size and weight. Make sure that your baby bag is easily accessible. If you are travelling during the day and the sun is bright, you may like to use a window shade to protect your baby. And don't forget to schedule stops for feeding and nappy changing. Most babies sleep well on a car journey so if you are going away you may prefer to drive at night when the chances are your baby will sleep through the journey.

Travelling by train

Train travel can be more relaxing for some and as long as you book ahead you will be guaranteed a seat.

Travelling by plane

This will take more planning. Your baby used to be able to travel on your passport but this is no longer the case so you will need to apply for a passport for your baby before you leave, if you are travelling abroad. You will also need to speak to your GP surgery about any possible vaccinations. As a general rule, breastfeeding mothers and their babies will both need to be vaccinated according to the recommendations of your destination, so check with your GP or travel clinic as to which vaccines your baby will need and the time frame over which they will have to be given.

If possible I think it is best to avoid countries where malaria is endemic. Some anti-malarial medication may be transmitted in breast milk but this won't provide enough protection so your baby will need his or her own medicines, and babies under two months old should not take anti-malarials. If you have to travel to a malaria zone you will need to be extra careful about protecting your baby from mosquito bites.

Check any age restrictions with your airline before you book – some airlines will accept babies over two days old while others will not allow your baby to fly until he or she is at least two weeks old. And some airlines will ask for a letter from your GP confirming that your baby is fit to fly. If you have had any medical complications or if your baby was born by caesarean section, there will also be restrictions on how soon you can fly so again, check with your airline before booking.

If you are breastfeeding, check with the airline as to whether you will be allowed to breastfeed on take off and landing. If you are bottle-feeding this can take a little more organizing. Airlines now only allow fluids up to 100 millilitres but if you are flying with your baby you will be allowed to carry larger volumes of expressed breast milk, formula milk, sterilized water or baby food. Airport staff may ask to open the containers.

At your destination be careful about the water you use for making up your baby's feeds. If you are bottle-feeding, you may need to use boiled bottled water rather than tap water. Make sure you check the labels as some bottled water has higher levels of salt and sulphate than is good for your baby. The salt (Na) content should be less than 200 milligrams (mg) per litre and the sulphate (SO or SO_4) should be less than 250 milligrams (mg) per litre.

6

Teething

A baby's first tooth is a memorable milestone, which happens at around six months for most children; although I have met babies who were born with a tooth already in place and some who still have no teeth on their first birthday.

Normal development

The first teeth to erupt are usually the lower two front teeth (the incisors) and if you are on the lookout, you will notice a pale swelling in the jaw just before the teeth break through. The next teeth to appear will be the upper incisors, followed by the teeth either side of these (the lateral incisors), and then the lower lateral incisors. Next, come the first molars in the upper jaw. These are the bigger teeth towards the back of the jaw and they are soon followed by the lower first molars at around 12–14 months. The upper canines come in around 16–18 months, followed by the lower canines and then the second molars in the lower jaw. The last teeth to erupt will be the second molars in the upper jaw. In all there are 20 milk teeth and they should all be through by the time your baby is two and a half years old.

Caring for your baby's teeth

Baby teeth help to guide the permanent teeth, which start to appear at about six years of age so it is important to look after them well. Get into the habit of cleaning them at least twice a day – decay in milk teeth can spread to the bone beneath and affect the health of the adult teeth. It's particularly important to clean teeth after the evening meal and before bedtime when your baby is weaned on to solids to ensure that no food particles are left in the mouth overnight. As he or she grows, your child may want to hold the toothbrush him- or herself and I think it's a good thing to encourage this but young children simply can't be expected to clean their teeth properly on their own, so you will need to finish the job and will probably need to supervise tooth brushing until your child is about seven years old.

I found the easiest way to clean teeth was to sit one child at a time on my lap with his or her back facing me. If your baby then fidgets and won't keep his or her head still you can rest your hand on baby's head to steady him or her. Use a soft-bristled brush and a tiny smear of toothpaste containing fluoride. Too much fluoride can cause fluorosis, a condition that discolours the teeth.

Teeth and diet

Healthy teeth need a diet rich in calcium and vitamin D, which your baby will get from dairy produce, oily fish and eggs. Your baby should also be having daily vitamin drops.

Sugar is harmful to teeth. Even tiny amounts of sugar in our diet can reduce the acidity of the mouth for half an hour at a time allowing dental decay. Wherever possible use savoury snacks and sugar-free drinks but if you are going to give sweet foods, give them all in one go. Frequent exposure to small amounts of sugar is more damaging than a single large dose.

Coping with teething

You will know when your baby is teething because he or she will dribble and will want to chew constantly. Baby's cheeks may look red and he or she may be irritable. Baby may also develop nappy rash but, contrary to popular belief, teething doesn't cause a temperature, vomiting or diarrhoea so don't dismiss these symptoms. As a general rule, the larger teeth at the back are likely to be more painful. All three of my children used a teething ring, which I kept cool in the fridge, and there are a variety of sugar-free teething gels available from chemists. Chewing on chilled carrots or an unsweetened rusk can be soothing, but never leave your baby unattended with food as a piece could break off and baby could choke. Protect your baby's delicate skin from becoming sore from dribbling by applying a barrier cream to his or her chin. If your child is in a lot of discomfort, don't be frightened to use sugar-free paracetamol liquid to keep your child pain free.

7

Developmental checks and milestones

Your baby will have a number of checks during his or her first year. Some of these will be done by your health visitor and some by your GP. Some will take place at your home, some in your GP surgery and some in a well baby clinic. It is important that you take your baby for these checks as they are a way of checking that he or she is healthy and developing normally. If there should be a problem it also means that this is picked up as early as possible and any treatment can be put in place quickly.

When your baby was born you will have been given a personal child health record, often referred to as the 'red book'. Every time your baby is weighed or measured, or has a developmental check or vaccination, the health care professionals will record the details in this book, so make sure you take it to all your appointments.

I will cover the vaccination schedule and the illnesses those vaccines protect against in Chapter 8, but below is a guideline to the checks you can expect your baby to have in the first year.

At birth

Your baby will be weighed at birth and again during the first week. It is completely normal for babies to lose a little weight in their first few days so don't panic. Most will regain their birth weight by day 14.

Day 1–3

A GP or midwife will examine your baby checking eyes, heart, hips and, for boys, testicles. I will explain in the 6–8-week check below, what they are looking for.

Day 5

Your baby will have a prick test to collect a few drops of blood to test for some rare diseases. Sometimes this test is done on day 6, 7 or 8. The diseases they are checking for include cystic fibrosis, sickle cell disease, congenital hypothyroidism and some rare inherited metabolic diseases (see Chapter 9).

Day 10–14

Your health visitor will do a review with you and your partner. This is an opportunity for you to discuss any concerns you may have and will allow your health visitor to offer you support with becoming a new parent.

Within 4–5 weeks

Your baby will have a routine hearing test within the first few weeks. If baby was born in hospital it may be done before you leave for home. It is a very quick test, which should cause no distress to your baby but it is important that it is done as 1 in 1,000 babies born in the UK are born deaf in one or both ears. If your baby spent more than 48 hours in a special care baby unit (SCBU) the incidence rises to 1 in 100. If a baby can't hear, it can have a significant impact on speech and language and social development so it is important that any problems are detected early. The test is called an automated acoustic emission test (AOAE). It involves placing a soft probe into your baby's ear. Quiet clicking sounds will then be sent through the probe and the sophisticated technology can tell if the inner ear (the cochlea) can hear those sounds. If your baby doesn't seem to be hearing, that doesn't automatically mean there is a problem. If baby is unsettled or has fluid in his or her ear or if there is background noise, this can affect the result and your team will arrange for a repeat test to be done.

6–8-week check

This is an important check up with your GP who will want to examine your baby and check on his or her development. It is also an opportunity for your GP to discuss any health promotion issues with you and for you to voice any concerns. Please don't be frightened to mention anything that is worrying you at this appointment. Becoming a new parent is daunting. At best your GP will be able to reassure you that everything is fine and at worst, if there is a potential problem, you and your baby will be offered the support and help that you need.

Let's start with the physical examination. Your baby may have already been weighed and measured (head to toe) and had the head circumference measured. This should then be plotted on a graph in your red book. Individual measurements are not particularly useful but if we plot your baby's measurements every time he or she is weighed and measured we can check that baby is thriving appropriately.

Your GP will also feel the soft spot (the fontanelle) in your baby's head and assess baby's general tone and colour. Your GP will shine a light into your baby's eyes looking for what is called a red reflex. The eye should appear red when this is done. If there are dark areas this could be due to a congenital cataract but if there is no red reflex in one eye at all this could be a very rare form of tumour called a retinoblastoma (see Chapter 9) and your GP would refer you urgently to the hospital to have further tests.

Your GP will also listen to your baby's heart looking for heart murmurs. If your baby has a 'hole in the heart', a defect in the septum between the chambers of the heart known as the atria and the ventricles, this can cause a murmur which may not be present at birth hence the need to recheck. Your GP will check your baby's lungs and abdomen and he or she will check the genitalia, particularly looking to confirm that both testicles are in the scrotum in boys. The testicles develop in the abdomen in the foetus and descend down into the scrotum. Undescended testicles can lead to future problems (see Chapter 9). Your GP will also check the skin creases in the thighs and do a special examination of the hips to check for hip dysplasia.

9 months – 1 year

During this time your baby will be reviewed again to check that he or she is developing normally and eating well and thriving. This is usually done by your health visitor.

How do I know if my baby is developing normally?

It's important to remember that all babies develop differently but below are a few rough guidelines as to when you can expect your baby to achieve certain milestones. It's important to remember that if your baby was born prematurely then we allow for that in terms of weight and development. So, if for example, your baby was born five weeks early then he or she may not do the sorts of things that the average 4-week-old baby would be doing until he or she is 9 weeks old. If your baby was very premature (less than 30 weeks), we continue to adjust for the first 2 years.

- *4 weeks*, your baby may start to focus on close up objects and seem to recognize faces. Baby will startle at sudden noises and, if you hold the baby above a surface, he or she will make reflex stepping movements.
- *4–6 weeks*, your baby may start to smile and make inarticulate sounds. Baby will start to lift his or her head and wriggle more.
- *3–4 months*, your baby will start to reach out and grab things. Baby may start to roll over and start to coo and babble. Baby will be able to focus on small objects and will turn towards quiet sounds. You may notice that if you lift baby up by the arms, he or she is starting to get more control of his or her head and that it doesn't lag behind so much.
- *6–7 months*, your baby should be ready to start solids now. Baby should be starting to sit up and able to pass things from hand to hand. Baby may also produce his or her first tooth.
- *9–10 months*, your baby may start to crawl and should be able to understand very simple commands, such as pointing at named objects or passing something to you. Baby may also start to develop a pincer (fingers and thumb) grip.
- *12 months,* this is when your baby may take his or her first steps and say his or her first words.

8

Vaccinations and the diseases they protect against

The childhood vaccination programme has expanded to include some new vaccines in recent years. It may feel a bit daunting to expose your baby to so many vaccinations and I am often asked whether a baby's immune system can cope with so many vaccines in the first year of life. The answer is absolutely yes. Our babies' immune systems are exposed to thousands of allergens and germs every day. What isn't safe is to leave them exposed to some very serious illnesses by delaying vaccination. I think it is easy to forget in modern day Britain just how devastating some of these illnesses can be, but believe me you only have to meet one child with post-measles encephalitis or who is totally deaf after meningitis and you will understand where I am coming from. To put my money where my mouth is – all three of my children had all their vaccines and I wouldn't do anything different if I was having my children now.

The vaccination schedule

As long as you have registered your baby with an NHS GP, you will automatically be sent appointments for these vaccinations. If you miss an appointment or can't make one, simply call your surgery and they will reschedule for you.

2 months

- 5-in-1 vaccine
- pneumococcal vaccine
- rotavirus vaccine
- meningitis B vaccine.

3 months

- 5-in-1 vaccine

- rotavirus vaccine
- meningitis C vaccine.

4 months

- 5-in-1 vaccine
- pneumococcal vaccine
- meningitis B vaccine.

12 months

- meningitis B vaccine – this is often given at the same time as the vaccines below.

12–13 months

- Hib/Men C booster
- pneumococcal vaccine
- MMR vaccine.

If my baby was premature should I postpone the vaccinations?

No. Premature babies are more vulnerable to infection so it is important that you take your baby as soon as you are called.

If my baby is unwell on the day of a vaccination appointment should I cancel?

If your baby has a cold but no fever it is fine for baby to still attend for his or her vaccines. If baby has a fever however it is best to telephone your surgery and postpone as the fever is likely to get worse with the vaccination.

Can I take my baby swimming before his or her vaccinations?

Yes. It is fine to take your baby swimming before any vaccinations.

The vaccinations

5-in-1 vaccine

The 5-in-1 vaccine is also sometimes referred to as the DTaP/IPV/Hib vaccine. It is given as a single injection usually into your baby's thigh. It protects against diphtheria, tetanus, whooping cough (pertussis), polio and haemophilus influenzae type B (Hib). It may cause your baby to be a little irritable that evening and he or she may have some redness around the injection site. There is no active ingredient in the vaccine so it is safe.

Pneumococcal vaccine

This is also given as an injection and may cause a mild fever, redness or hardness at the site of injection.

Rotavirus vaccine

This is given by liquid dropper directly into the mouth. The vaccine contains a weakened form of the vaccine, which is not strong enough to cause infection but is strong enough to trigger the immune system to develop immunity to future rotavirus infections. Since its introduction we have seen a 70 per cent fall in the cases of rotavirus.

Meningitis B vaccine

This is also given by injection. It is made from three proteins found on the surface of the meningitis B bacteria. It has no active ingredient so it cannot cause meningitis. It may cause a fever 24 hours after vaccination and some redness at the injection site. Your baby may also be slightly irritable for a short period.

Meningitis C vaccine

This is made using part of the surface of the meningitis C vaccine so again is very safe. It may cause redness at the site of infection and fever and occasionally babies may vomit after the injection. It was introduced in 1999 and amazingly meningitis C is virtually eradicated from this country as a result!

Hib/Men C booster

Again this is an inactivated vaccine designed to boost immunity to these infections in your baby's future.

MMR vaccine

This vaccine contains weakened versions of the viruses that cause measles, mumps and rubella. Thousands of column inches have been written about a possible link with this vaccine and autism but despite multiple research projects, no link has ever been found. Autism is of course a disorder of communication and socialization so it inevitably starts to present at a time when your child begins to speak and communicate, which is when we give the vaccine. I am totally happy that there is no link and as I have said all three of my children had both doses of the MMR and I would do the same today.

I am often asked about the possibility of single vaccines, namely giving the measles, mumps and rubella vaccines separately. These vaccines are not licensed here in the UK and have to be given some time apart so you simply run the risk of leaving your child exposed to these viruses for longer. The MMR can cause swollen glands for a couple of days and a measles-like rash for up to three days but these are not contagious.

The illnesses we vaccinate against

Diphtheria

Diphtheria is a highly contagious and potentially fatal condition caused by bacteria spread via coughs and sneezes and by contact with infected people or their clothing. Thanks to the vaccination programme it is now very rare in Britain. Symptoms include a high fever (38 degrees or more), a sore throat with a thick greyish coating at the back of the throat and problems breathing. It is usually diagnosed with a swab test and needs urgent treatment with antibiotics to prevent potential complications affecting the heart and nervous system.

Tetanus

Tetanus is caused by bacteria getting into a wound. It is a serious and potentially fatal condition but is now very rare because of the vaccination schedule. I have only ever seen one case of tetanus in my clinical career and that was when I was working in outback Australia, where I looked after an Aboriginal man who developed tetanus after the tribal doctor had been packing his leg wound with dried camel dung. The symptoms of tetanus include a high fever, rapid heartbeat, sweating and stiffness of the muscles of the jaw, sometimes referred to as lockjaw. There are often also painful muscle spasms elsewhere in the body. It is treated with tetanus immunoglobulin and antibiotics. Patients often need admitting to intensive care.

Whooping cough (pertussis)

Whooping cough is another highly contagious disease which causes the characteristic 'whoop' sound as the individual breathes in after coughing. The early symptoms may seem like any other cough or cold but as they develop the cough becomes more severe and patients often cough up thick phlegm. Young babies under six months old may not make the whoop sound but you may notice them gagging after coughing bouts or they may even look like they have stopped breathing. The cough can last for three months and is treated with antibiotics.

Polio

Polio is now eradicated from the UK due to the very successful vaccination programme and is likely to be eradicated globally in years to come. It is caused by a picornavirus, which is one of a group of viruses that live in the gut. In fact the virus can be detected in the stools of a polio sufferer up to six weeks after the start of the illness. Around 95 per cent of cases are mild with no symptoms or there may be a mild viral illness, but more serious cases affect the brain and spinal cord. In this instance the individual will develop a high fever, headache and stiff neck and there may be progressive weakness or even paralysis of the limbs and breathing difficulties if the muscles of the chest wall are involved. There is no specific treatment for polio, which is why it is so important to be vaccinated.

Haemophilus influenzae type B infections

Haemophilus influenzae type B is a bacteria that can cause a number of different problems, including meningitis, pneumonia and septicaemia (blood poisoning). It is a very serious infection – 1 in every 20 children who develop Hib meningitis don't survive and many of those who do can be left with deafness, learning disabilities and epilepsy. Hib is spread in the same way as coughs and colds but is thankfully rare in the UK since the Hib vaccination was included in the childhood vaccination programme in 1992.

Pneumococcal infections

These are caused by a bacteria which can cause a wide variety of infections, the most serious being blood poisoning, pneumonia, meningitis and infections of the bones (osteomyelitis) and joints (septic arthritis).

Rotavirus infections

Rotavirus is highly infectious and is easily spread among families. The virus can also survive for several days on surfaces so personal and home hygiene are crucial if your household is affected. It can cause profuse diarrhoea, which can lead to dehydration.

Meningitis B and C infection

Meningitis is infection of the membranes that cover the brain (the meninges). It presents with a high fever, but cold hands and feet. Babies may be floppy and listless and off their food. There may be a high-pitched cry and the skin may look blotchy. It is a medical emergency and needs hospital treatment with antibiotics urgently. About a quarter of children who develop bacterial meningitis will have long-term problems such as hearing loss after the infection.

Measles

Measles is a highly contagious viral infection. Symptoms usually develop ten days after the initial infection and start with cold-like symptoms. Sufferers go on to develop sore red eyes and may be sensitive to light. They can have a very high temperature (up to 40 degrees) and they develop white-greyish spots on the inside of the cheeks. These are called koplik spots. A few days later the classic pink-brown blotchy rash appears. It starts on the head or neck and spreads across the body. Sadly, there are some serious complications associated with measles including meningitis, seizures, hepatitis and blindness. There is a very rare but fatal long-term problem affecting 1 in 25,000 cases where the brain becomes fatally inflamed several years after the initial infection.

Mumps

Mumps is a viral infection causing swelling of the parotid glands, which are glands found at the side of the face just in front of the ears. Sufferers may also get a high fever and joint pains. It can also cause swelling of the testicles in boys and the ovaries in girls. Very rarely it can cause a form of meningitis.

Rubella

Rubella is another viral infection that can cause a high fever, cold-like symptoms, aching joints, swollen glands and a pink spotty rash. It is spread in the same way as coughs and colds.

If a pregnant woman contracts rubella it can have very serious consequences for the unborn baby including blindness, deafness, brain damage and heart abnormalities.

We are very lucky in this country to have such an effective child-hood vaccination programme. I hope I have persuaded you to use it.

9

A to Z of infant ailments

Balanitis

Balanitis is inflammation of the head of the penis, causing redness, soreness and swelling at the tip of the penis. There may also be a rash further down the penis. It can happen in babies, older boys and adults, but in young babies it is most commonly associated with infrequent nappy changing. The urine contained within the nappy acts as an irritant so it is important to change nappies regularly and avoid other potential irritants such as bubble baths and soaps. It is most commonly treated by avoiding the irritants. Steroid, antibiotic and antifungal creams may also be needed.

Birthmarks

Birthmarks are areas of pigmented skin or a collection of blood vessels in the skin. They are not always present at birth and may develop within the first few months of life. There are several types.

- *Brown birthmarks*, these are also called moles and are permanent.
- *Stork marks*, these derived their name from the fact that they appear on the back of the neck and the forehead so were said to have been left by the stork after delivering the baby! These will fade and completely disappear in the first few years.
- *Mongolian blue spots*, these are found on the lower back or buttocks in darker-skinned babies and have in the past been mistaken for bruises.
- *Strawberry naevus*, this is a raised pink or red mark, which may have a dimpled surface like that of a strawberry. It or they can be quite large and parents sometimes find them unsightly, particularly as they often get bigger and change colour before they disappear. Unless they are impairing vision we try not to treat

them as they rarely cause any problem to the child and they will resolve by the age of five without treatment.

- *Port wine stain*, this is often a larger sometimes red or purple birthmark, which can become more raised over time. They are twice as common in girls as they are in boys. They can sometimes be part of a syndrome such as Sturge–Weber syndrome, which is associated with epilepsy, or Klippel–Trenaunay syndrome, which is associated with overgrowth of a limb, or Proteus syndrome, also associated with overgrowth of bone, skin and other tissues. These are rare syndromes and need to be managed by a specialist. Your GP may recommend that your baby has specialist laser treatment to treat a port wine stain.

Blocked tear ducts

Babies can sometimes be born with an underdeveloped tear duct system. The good news is that 90 per cent of them will have corrected without the need for surgical intervention. The baby may appear to have watery eyes and may develop a discharge. Your GP will show you how to massage the eye to encourage drainage. Persistent cases may need a small operation under anaesthetic to probe the tear duct and open it up.

Bronchiolitis

Bronchiolitis is an infection of the small airways (the bronchioles) in babies and children under two. The condition usually starts with a runny nose and cough so may seem just like a cold but then goes on to be associated with a high fever, difficulty feeding and rapid or noisy breathing. In severe cases the baby may look blue around the mouth and really struggle with breathing. This is a medical emergency.

Bronchiolitis is caused by a virus called the respiratory syncytial virus (RSV). It affects around one in three children in their first year, especially during the winter. Thankfully, most can be cared for at home but about 2–3 per cent of babies will need to be admitted to hospital. Treatment includes keeping the air moist. A humidifier is great for this or, if you have radiators on, put warm wet towels on them to encourage moisture into the air. Make sure you keep your baby well hydrated and try to nurse baby slightly upright to make his or her breathing easier. It is important that you don't smoke around your baby and that you use paracetamol or ibuprofen to control the fever. (Paracetamol can be given to babies over two months old and ibuprofen to those over three months and weighing at least 5 kilograms.) Saline nasal drops may also help clear the airways. In more severe cases, your baby may need to be admitted to hospital and may need to be given extra oxygen.

You can protect your baby from bronchiolitis by being vigilant about handwashing and keeping surfaces and toys clean. The virus can live outside the human body for several hours. Also try to avoid taking your baby to see people with coughs and colds.

Cataracts

Cataracts are areas of cloudiness in the lens of the eye that mean vision becomes blurred. We tend to think of them most frequently as something that is associated with old age but some babies are born with what is called congenital cataracts and some develop them in the first six months of life – these are called infantile cataracts.

If only one eye is affected there is unlikely to be an obvious cause but when both eyes are affected (bilateral cataracts), they are more likely to run in the family. They can also be associated with rubella if the mother was affected when the baby was developing in the womb. If your health visitor or GP notices a cataract, he or she will refer your baby to an ophthalmologist who will tell you whether surgery is needed to remove the cataract.

Chickenpox

Chickenpox is caused by the varicella-zoster virus. Most children will have had chickenpox before leaving primary school. Your baby may be off colour with a fever and loss of appetite for a few days before the classic spots develop. They tend to form in clusters anywhere on the body. The spots start as small itchy red spots, which then blister and, after a couple of days, they crust over. Chickenpox is infectious from a couple of days before the rash develops until the last spot has crusted over, which is usually about five or six days. You should keep your baby away from pregnant women or anyone with a weakened immune system (such as people receiving chemotherapy) during this time. There is no specific treatment for chickenpox so it is a case of easing your baby's symptoms with paracetamol, calamine lotion and cooling gels until he or she recovers. Unlike most viruses, chickenpox never completely clears from the body. After the infection it crawls back up the nerve endings and goes to sleep but later in life, particularly if you are very run down, it can reactivate, causing shingles.

Colic

Infantile colic is common, affecting as many as one in five babies. It usually starts at just a few weeks old, lasting until the baby is four months old and occasionally six months. It causes huge distress to parents, not least because they are sleep deprived as a result. Typical symptoms include intense bouts of crying that can last several hours. Colicky babies will be thriving in terms of weight but will often look in pain as they clench their fists and draw their knees up to the chest. I have met many utterly exhausted parents of colicky babies and the most important things for you to know if your baby has colic is that it will get better, that it isn't anything you have or haven't done and that, as awful as it looks, it is distressing you more than your baby.

Try to make sure you burp your baby after feeds and feed baby in a more upright position to stop baby swallowing air. A warm bath and gentle massage to the tummy may help. You can also speak to your health visitor or pharmacist about drops to add to feeds in bottle-fed babies.

Congenital hypothyroidism

This is rare, affecting about 1 in 3,500 newborn babies, but it is a serious condition and that is why it is one of the conditions we check for in the heel prick test (see Chapter 7). The thyroid gland is like the engine in a car. The thyroid gland produces the hormone thyroxine, which drives our metabolism. Without it we die, which is why we test every baby in the UK for hypothyroidism. If the heel prick test suggests your baby could have congenital hypothyroidism your doctors will want to do other tests to confirm the diagnosis and will arrange a painless scan of your baby's neck to check whether the thyroid gland is present. Some types of hypothyroidism can run in families so your doctors will talk to you about any risks for future babies. Once diagnosed your baby will need daily medication to replace thyroxine and regular blood tests to monitor the dose needed. Most babies born with congenital hypothyroidism will grow up healthily, but a small number may have additional problems such as hearing problems and learning difficulties.

Conjunctivitis

Conjunctivitis simply means inflammation (*itis*) of the white part of the eye (the conjunctiva). It can be caused by bacteria, viruses, irritants and allergies. Newborn babies are particularly prone to bacterial infection as they pass through the birth canal, causing a discharge and red eyes. If your GP or midwife suspects conjunctivitis, he or she will take a swab test from your baby's eye and suggest antibiotic drops or ointment.

Constipation

As I have said many times before, babies are very individual but, as a rough guide, babies under the age of four months may pass a motion three to four times a day. When solids are introduced this will reduce such that, when a baby is fully weaned, baby is likely to be having nearer to one motion a day. The important thing is that your baby shouldn't be straining to pass a motion. Constipation is rare in babies on a purely liquid diet, although it is slightly more common in exclusively bottle-fed babies than it is in breastfed babies. If your baby is passing very solid motions and appears in discomfort when his or her bowels are open, you may want to add drinks of water between feeds. Increase the fluids this way rather than diluting the formula milk. If baby has started solids, you should look to increase the fibre in the diet by increasing fruit and vegetables. If this doesn't work, speak to your GP about which are the best laxatives to use in an infant. We prefer to use stool softeners or osmotic laxatives rather than stimulant laxatives.

Cradle cap

Cradle cap is the term used for the yellowish scales and plaques that form on a baby's scalp. It usually causes no distress to the child but lots of concern from worried parents. It starts within the first couple of months of life and will resolve within your baby's first year. We don't really know why it happens but one theory is that it is linked to maternal hormones that are still circulating in the infant. Try not to pick at the scales as this may cause irritation to the delicate underlying skin. You can try massaging almond or olive oil into the scalp to loosen the scales. You can also buy special cradle cap shampoos from the chemist.

Croup

Croup is a viral infection of the airways that develops the characteristic barking cough and harsh sound as the child breathes in – this is called stridor. Symptoms are often worse at night and usually only last a few days before improving but can last for a couple of weeks. Most young children can be looked after at home but some babies become very ill with a high fever, severe breathing difficulties and a blue tinge to their lips or become very drowsy and these children need to be admitted to hospital. Croup occurs mostly at around one year of age but it can affect children from six months and occasionally even as young as three months. Treatment is similar to that for bronchiolitis (see above) but your GP may also give your baby a dose of steroids to reduce any swelling in the throat and ease his or her breathing.

General hygiene measures such as hand washing and cleaning surfaces and toys will help prevent the spread of croup and it is important that you take your baby for the routine vaccinations as some of the viruses we vaccinate against, such as measles, mumps, rubella, diphtheria, tetanus, whooping cough, polio and haemophilus influenzae type B, can cause croup.

Cystic fibrosis

Cystic fibrosis is an inherited condition where the lungs and digestive system get bunged up with sticky mucus. One in 2,500 babies born in the UK are affected. It is one of the conditions screened for at birth with the heel prick test. In the past, children with cystic fibrosis invariably died young (often in their teens or early twenties) but with improved treatment and earlier diagnosis a baby born with cystic fibrosis today could expect to live until 50.

Treatment includes regular physiotherapy to help drain the excess mucus from the chest, antibiotics to treat infections and medicines to help clear the airways. Some patients with cystic fibrosis will also have diabetes and need insulin injections. Most people with diabetes are told to watch their calorie intake but this is not the case with cystic fibrosis. They need a diet high in calories and rich in fat and protein as they need to maintain weight so that they are strong enough to fight infection. The condition can affect the production of enzymes in the pancreas that aid digestion, so cystic fibrosis sufferers often need to take extra digestive enzymes to ensure they can extract the nutrients from their food. It is also important that anyone with cystic fibrosis has a flu jab every year.

If a baby is diagnosed with cystic fibrosis, he or she may need extra salt, as salt is lost through the skin with cystic fibrosis, but this is something that should be done under the supervision of cystic fibrosis specialists. Don't ever be tempted to add it yourself.

Dehydration

Dehydration occurs when your body loses more fluid than you take in. Older children will be able to tell you they are thirsty but if your baby has had diarrhoea or vomiting or hasn't been taking fluids, you will need to look out for the signs of dehydration. These include there being fewer or no wet nappies, the soft spot on the top of the head (the fontanelle) feeling a bit sunken in, having no tears when they cry or just being uncharacteristically drowsy. Doctors also look for something called skin turgor. If you gently pinch the skin on the back of your baby's hand it should fall back into place immediately you let go. If it looks tented for a while this could be a sign of dehydration. If you are in any doubt, get your baby checked by a doctor, but like all things, prevention is better than cure so make sure you are on the lookout and if your baby is at risk, offer bottles of water as well as feeds.

Diarrhoea

An occasional loose stool is common in babies but if your baby suddenly develops persistently loose stools, he or she has diarrhoea. The most common cause is a viral infection, which typically will last five to seven days. It can also be caused by bacterial infection or by parasites spread from people around them and is why we are so keen on hygiene around babies. Most cases of diarrhoea can be managed at home but you should seek medical help if your baby is showing signs of dehydration (see above).

Eczema

Eczema is very common in babies, particularly if other members of the family have suffered with eczema, asthma and hayfever. Typically the red scaly patches affect the face, neck, behind the ears and the creases of the elbows and knees but eczema can occur any-where on the body. Eczema is basically a combination of dryness and inflammation in the skin. Make sure you keep your baby's skin well hydrated with an emollient from your GP or pharmacist and apply the emollient with downward strokes. Avoid anything per-fumed as this can dry the skin more and apply the emollient with downward strokes and avoid any soaps, bubble baths or aqueous cream as these can also aggravate the problem. Avoid man-made fabrics if you can and stick to cotton clothing and bed linen. Try to maintain a constant room temperature, which is not too hot or too cold as both extremes can cause eczema to flare. If the skin is looking very red, you may need steroid creams from your GP. Parents are often worried about this but your GP will advise you how to use the cream and it is better that your baby is comfortable. As your baby grows you will need to keep his or her finger nails short to stop baby from scratching the skin. Fortunately for most babies, eczema does improve over time.

Hip dysplasia

Hip dysplasia is an abnormality of the hip that is usually present from birth such that the hip joint isn't as secure and stable as it should be. About 80 per cent of cases occur in girls and it is more common if someone else in the family has had the problem, although interestingly it is also more common in the firstborn child. It can also be more common if the baby was in the breech position (feet or bottom down) in the womb.

Hip dysplasia is checked for in the baby checks described in Chapter 7. In particular doctors are looking for asymmetrical skin creases in the thighs and for any clicking in the hip when it is examined.

If your GP suspects hip dysplasia, an ultrasound scan will be arranged. In older babies (over four months), your GP may arrange an X-ray. If hip dysplasia is confirmed then you will probably be given a special harness for your baby to wear permanently for six weeks. In children over six months or in those for whom the harness is not successful, your baby may need a general anaesthetic so that the doctors can put the hip into the correct position and then place a plaster cast around it to keep it in place for 12 weeks. Very rarely, if none of this works, your child may need an operation to loosen the tendons and strengthen the joint. It can be an ordeal going through all this but the good news is that the outlook is excellent if children are diagnosed and treatment started before six months of age.

Intussusception

Intussusception is a serious condition where part of the bowel telescopes inside another part like a finger in a glove being turned inside out. We don't really know why it happens but it is more common in the winter months so one theory is that it could be triggered by a virus. It is most common in boys under a year old and can come on quite suddenly. So, a child who seemed previously well may cry out and may pull his or her knees up to his or her chest. This pain may come in spasms every 15 to 20 minutes. Bowel movements may alter, with some babies developing diarrhoea and others constipation. If you notice your baby's stools look like redcurrant jelly then this must be checked out. If left untreated, the blood supply to the bowel may be cut off and the bowel could die so it is important that you see a doctor immediately if you suspect intussusception. The doctor may be able to reverse the intussusception with a barium or air enema which simply uses gentle pressure but if this doesn't work, your baby will need an operation to free the portion of bowel that is trapped.

Lactose intolerance

Most formula milks are prepared from cow's milk. It is possible that your baby could develop an intolerance to the protein in formula. Typical symptoms include diarrhoea, vomiting, bloating and excess wind. If your GP thinks your baby may have a lactose intolerance or allergy, he or she may suggest a special formula that has been fully hydrolysed. By that we mean the proteins are broken down into much smaller parts so are less allergenic. You can buy partially hydrolysed formula milk in the shops but if you suspect a problem, talk to your GP who can advise on the best formula. Don't be tempted to opt for goat's milk formula unless specifically advised to do so by your GP as there can be crossover between sensitivity to cow's milk and goat's milk proteins.

Milia

Milia are tiny white spots that appear across a baby's nose, cheeks or chin. They usually disappear on their own after a month or two so don't need any treatment. They don't bother the baby at all and have no long-term complications so it is well to leave them alone until they heal on their own.

Nappy rash

Nappy rash is very common. It is caused by chafing or rubbing or by the sensitive skin being in contact with urine and faeces for too long, which is why it is important to check your baby's nappy regularly and change it when soiled or wet and ensure the skin is clean and dry, paying special attention to all the skin creases before putting on a new nappy. If you can, let your baby's bottom get some air from time to time too. If your baby is prone to nappy rash you may like to use a zinc-based barrier cream to protect baby's skin. Most nappy rash problems can be managed at home but if there is severe inflammation, check with your GP as you may need a different cream to treat it.

Posseting

See Vomiting.

Pyloric stenosis

The exit from the stomach to the small bowel is made up of muscle and is called the pylorus. In some babies this muscle is thicker than usual, making it more difficult for food to pass into the small bowel. This means these babies are more prone to vomiting after feeds and within days they develop what is called projectile vomiting. This is completely different from the sort of overspill that is posseting. The vomit may travel several feet. Symptoms start to develop around six weeks old and it is more common in boys than it is in girls.

If your GP suspects pyloric stenosis, you may be asked to feed your baby in front of him or her. Your GP will be looking for a hard lump of muscle on the right side of your baby's stomach, which is the pylorus straining. Your GP may also want to arrange a scan to look at the muscle. If pyloric stenosis is confirmed, your baby will need an operation under general anaesthetic, which is daunting I know but it is a simple operation and only lasts about 30 minutes after which your baby should make a rapid recovery.

Retinoblastoma

A retinoblastoma is a very rare form of cancer of the retina at the back of the eye. It affects children under five years old. It is why we check for the red reflex in babies (see Chapter 7). Of children who have this condition, 98 per cent will be cured if the condition is picked up early. It can be linked to a faulty gene so if someone in your family has had a retinoblastoma your doctors may want to check your baby's eyes more frequently than usual. If a retinoblastoma is diagnosed, treatment may involve laser treatment or the application of heat (thermotherapy) or freezing the tumour (cryotherapy). Very rarely, if there is a large tumour, your child will need surgery to remove the eye.

Sickle cell disease

Sickle cell disease is another disease that is checked for with the heel prick test. It affects mainly African, Caribbean, Middle Eastern, Asian and Eastern Mediterranean people. The condition is associated with abnormally shaped blood cells, which affects the ability of the body to transport oxygen effectively. The blood cells also don't live as long and it is difficult to reproduce blood cells quickly enough so that patients become anaemic.

If your child is diagnosed, you will be referred to a specialist team, which could include haematologists (specialists in disorders of the blood), paediatricians (specialists in children's medicine), physiotherapists and clinical psychologists.

Because the blood cells are an abnormal shape they can get clogged in the blood vessels, which is very painful. This is called a sickle cell crisis and the team looking after you will give you advice on how to avoid crises such as drinking plenty of water, taking regular exercise, eating well and avoiding triggers such as stress, extremes of temperature and high altitudes.

Squint

A squint is where the eyes don't look in the same direction. Most commonly, one eye looks in but it can also mean an eye looks out, up or down. It is normal for this to happen in children up to about 12 weeks of age but 1 in 20 children has a squint that persists after three months. If you notice this in your child mention it to your health visitor or take your child to your GP who will arrange for him or her to be assessed by an optometrist. A squint usually occurs because one eye is significantly stronger than the other and the optometrist will probably suggest using patches to cover the stronger eye for a short while each day. This will encourage the brain to concentrate on the messages from the squinting eye and improve the vision in that eye. Patching won't correct the appearance of the squint though and your child may need an operation at some point to straighten the eye.

Undescended testicles

Testicles develop in the abdomen when little boys are growing in the womb and they are supposed to descend down into the scrotum about a month or two before birth. About 1 in 25 boys are born with one or both testicles not yet in the scrotal sac. This is something that will be checked for in your baby checks. Initially your doctors will probably keep an eye on things in the hope that the testicles will move down within the first six months of life but if at six months they are still undescended, your GP will refer you to a specialist to consider an operation to bring the testicle down into the scrotum. This is called an orchidopexy and is relatively straightforward. It is important it is done though as testes that stay in the abdomen may not produce healthy sperm, which could lead to fertility problems later in life and there is a slightly increased risk of testicular cancer if the operation is not done.

Vomiting

Babies often bring up a little milk after a feed. This is called posseting and is nothing to worry about. It often looks more significant than it is and I have met lots of mums concerned that their baby simply can't be getting enough milk. If you take a tea towel and pour a small amount of milk on to it, you will be amazed just how far it can spread! That is why it looks more worrying than it is. To be sure, get your baby weighed regularly – if he or she is gaining weight appropriately then your baby is getting enough nutrition. If the vomiting is more serious than this in young children it is likely to be part of an infective illness. The most important thing you can do is to keep your baby well hydrated (see Dehydration). If you are in doubt and concerned that your baby is becoming listless, has a high fever and won't take a feed, get baby checked out immediately.

10

Your baby's medicine cabinet

I have always said that from the moment your baby is born (or actually from the moment of your first positive pregnancy test!) you will have two words tattooed through you like a stick of rock and they are 'guilty' and 'worried'. This goes with the job description, but along with it go some of the most wonderful experiences life can give you. Of course, you can't be prepared for every eventuality but it is a good idea to have a basic medicine cabinet to cover minor ailments. Below is a list of what I would recommend you keep to hand:

- infant paracetamol – I'm not sure how I would have got through my babies' first years without it!
- infant ibuprofen
- a digital thermometer
- calamine lotion
- barrier cream for nappy areas
- saline drops for blocked noses
- baby nail scissors or nail clippers
- baby sunscreen
- baby safe insect repellent
- cotton wool balls
- syringe for administering medicine – you may find this easier than using a dropper or a spoon.

11

First aid for babies

Of course we all hope that we won't need the advice given in this chapter but it's worth being familiar with what's in here so that you will know what to do if your baby is in need of first aid help or you are in a situation where someone else's child needs immediate treatment.

Burns

Baby skin is very delicate. Even a warm cup of coffee could cause a burn so if your baby has been in contact with something hot, run the skin under cold water for at least ten minutes and then apply cling film to the area. If you are concerned, take your baby to the accident and emergency department of a hospital where staff can dress it with special burns dressings and assess whether anything more needs to be done.

Choking

If your baby appears to be choking hold baby face down across your lap with baby's head lower than his or her bottom and, using the heel of your hand, give five firm blows to baby's back. If this doesn't dislodge whatever he or she is choking on, try turning baby over and, using two fingers, press inward and upward in the middle of the chest just below the nipples. You can repeat this cycle but if the symptoms are not resolving or if your baby is looking blue, call 999 immediately.

Fever

All children will get a fever at some point. If your child has a fever, take layers of clothing off and give baby the recommended dose of ibuprofen or paracetamol. You could also try giving baby a tepid bath and cool fluids.

Head injury

The first time your baby rolls over or takes the first step is such an exciting moment but I know it has taken some families by surprise. It is important not to leave your baby unattended, but it can happen that in a split second baby may move and bash his or her head. If your baby has a bump, apply something cold to the injury, such as frozen vegetables wrapped in a tea towel, and comfort the baby. If baby becomes drowsy or vomits, get him or her to a doctor.

Seizures

If your baby has a seizure check the area around, making sure that you move any furniture or objects that babies could injure themselves on, but do not restrain your baby. When the seizure has settled remove any excess clothing if you suspect a fever fit and give medication to reduce a fever as soon as he or she is able to take it safely. If this is the first fit, seek medical advice.

The unconscious child

If you should find your baby unconscious, check for breathing. If your baby is breathing, support baby on his or her side with baby's head slightly below his or her bottom so that the airway stays open and call 999. If your baby is not breathing, shout for help, asking someone to call 999 while you tilt baby's head back by placing one hand on baby's forehead and one finger of the other hand under baby's chin. Then, cover baby's nose and mouth with yours and blow five breaths into baby. Then, push firmly with two fingers into the middle of the chest 30 times before giving baby another two breaths and then more compressions and keep doing this until help arrives.

12

Safety in and around the home

There are a few things that you need to do to ensure that your baby's environment is as safe as possible and what you need to do will change as your baby grows and starts to explore his or her own environment. We used to laugh that we could guess the ages of our friends' children when we visited their houses by the height of their ornaments! Here are a few of my top tips for household safety.

- Make sure you have smoke alarms and carbon monoxide alarms fitted.
- Have a fire extinguisher and fire blanket in the house.
- When your baby starts to explore by crawling, shuffling or walking you will need to ensure that all cupboard doors have child safety catches on them.
- Fill all electric sockets with dummy plugs.
- Make sure that all windows are securely shut and check there isn't furniture around that a child could climb on to to access any windows.
- Keep all pet bowls clean and out of reach where possible.
- Use a safety film on any glass doors that your child could fall against when he or she starts walking.
- Make sure that all electrical cords are out of reach.
- Don't leave hot liquids where your child could reach them.
- Don't use table cloths – even a crawling baby could tug on a table cloth and cause damage.
- Don't have self-closing doors that could trap a baby's hand.
- Be careful about lightweight furniture, which your baby could use to pull on to try to stand up.
- Use a non-slip bath mat.
- Install a stair gate before you think you may need it!

12

Safety in and around the home

Index